FOGSI EEBR 2025

Ethical Evidence-Based Recommendations

# Endometriosis

## Disclaimer

This Ethical Evidence-Based Recommendation (EEBR) document is drafted following a consensus between esteemed FOGSI experts and stakeholders and are based on the scientific evidence available at the time of preparation.

EEBRs should be used for information and educational purposes. They do not replace the need for application of clinical judgment to each individual presentation, or variations based on individual patient and resource setting.

Furthermore, EEBRs do not constitute or imply the endorsement of any of the included technologies, therapies, or techniques by FOGSI.

# FOGSI EEBR 2025
# Ethical Evidence-Based Recommendations
# Endometriosis


*Editor-in-Chief*

**Sunita Tandulwadkar**
MD (Obs and Gyne) FICS (Gyne-Endoscopy) FICOG
President, FOGSI (2025–2026)
Gynecological Endoscopist and ART & IVF Specialist
Head, Department of Obstetrics and Gynecology
Chief, IVF & Endoscopy Center, Ruby Hall Clinic, Pune
Founder and Medical Director
Solo Clinic IVF—A Center for Excellence in Infertility and Endoscopy, Pune
Founder and Medical Director
Solo Stem Cells—A Stem Cell Research and Application Center, Pune
Founder and Director, Alive Regenerative Wellness, Pune, Maharashtra, India

*Editors*

**Pankaj Talwar** MD PhD
Director at i-Ceat | i-Consult| i-HOMaa
Dean
Department of Clinical Embryology and Reproductive Sciences
Shridhar University
Pilani, Rajasthan, India
i-HOMaa Fertility Clinic
Gurugram, Haryana, India
President, Indian Fertility Society (2024–2026)

**Pratik Tambe**
MD FICOG FICRM FICMCH FIAOG
ART Consultant, Gynec Endoscopic Surgeon
Department of Obstetrics and Gynecology
Reproductive Medicine, Gynec Endoscopic Surgery
High Risk Pregnancy
Ashirwad IVF
Mumbai, Maharashtra, India
Governing Council Member, ICOG and ICRM
Managing Committee Member, MOGS, ISAR, MSR
Past Chair, FOGSI and AMOGS Endocrinology Committees

*Experts*

**Rishma Pai**
MD FRCOG DNB FCPS FICOG
Consultant Gynecologist and Infertility Specialist
Department of Obstetrics and Gynecology, IVF
Lilavati, Jaslok, and Hinduja Hospitals
Mumbai, Maharashtra, India
Treasurer, International Federation of Fertility Societies (IFFS)
Former President, FOGSI, ISAR, IAGE
Member, FIGO Menstrual Disorders Committee

**Nandita Palshetkar**
MD FCPS FICOG FRCOG (UK)
Professor Emeritus
Department of Obstetrics and Gynecology
DY Patil School of Medicine, Navi Mumbai
Infertility Specialist
Lilavati Hospital IVF Center, Mumbai, Maharashtra, India
Scientific Director and Co-Founder
Bloom IVF and BAUFICI Genetics
President, Indian Society for Assisted Reproduction (2022–2024)
President, Association of Maharashtra Obstetric and Gynaecological Societies (2020–2022)
Past President, FOGSI, IAGE, MOGS and MSR

*Convener*

**Pooja Lodha** DNB (Obs and Gyne)
Fellow, Fetal Medicine, FOGSI-FMF UK Certified
Lead Consultant
Department of Fetal Medicine
Ruby Hall Clinic and Bharati Vidyapeeth University and Hospital, Pune
Director, Kangaroo Cradle, Fetal Care Centre
Pune, Maharashtra, India



JAYPEE

**JAYPEE BROTHERS MEDICAL PUBLISHERS**
*The Health Sciences Publisher*
**New Delhi | London**

**Jaypee Brothers Medical Publishers (P) Ltd**

**Headquarters**
Jaypee Brothers Medical Publishers (P) Ltd
EMCA House, 23/23-B
Ansari Road, Daryaganj
New Delhi 110 002, India
Landline: +91-11-23272143, +91-11-23272703
+91-11-23282021, +91-11-23245672
Email: jaypee@jaypeebrothers.com

**Corporate Office**
Jaypee Brothers Medical Publishers (P) Ltd
4838/24, Ansari Road, Daryaganj
New Delhi 110 002, India
Phone: +91-11-43574357
Fax: +91-11-43574314
Email: jaypee@jaypeebrothers.com

**Overseas Office**
JP Medical Ltd.
83, Victoria Street, London
SW1H 0HW (UK)
Phone: +44 20 3170 8910
Fax: +44 (0)20 3008 6180
Email: info@jpmedpub.com

Website: www.jaypeebrothers.com
Website: www.jaypeedigital.com



**Inquiries for bulk sales may be solicited at:** jaypee@jaypeebrothers.com

***FOGSI EEBR 2025—Ethical Evidence-Based Recommendations: Endometriosis***

*First Edition:* **2025**

ISBN: 978-93-6616-746-6

*Printed in India*

# Contributors

**Bindu Bajaj**
MD PGCC (Hospital Management)
Professor and Head
Department of Obstetrics and Gynecology
Vardhman Mahavir Medical College and Safdarjung Hospital
New Delhi, India

**Harpreet Kaur**
MD DNB FNB (Reproductive Medicine) MRCOG (UK)
Associate Professor
Department of Obstetrics and Gynecology
All India Institute of Medical Sciences
Bilaspur, Himachal Pradesh, India

**Maansi Jain**
MBBS MS (Obs and Gyne) Diploma Clinical ART Fellowship in Reproductive Medicine and Surgery (Singapore)
Consultant
Department of Reproductive Medicine and Endoscopic Surgery
KJIVF and Laparoscopy Center
New Delhi, India

**Nandita Palshetkar**
MD FCPS FICOG FRCOG (UK)
Professor Emeritus
Department of Obstetrics and Gynecology
DY Patil School of Medicine
Navi Mumbai, Maharashtra, India
Infertility Specialist
Lilavati Hospital IVF Center, Mumbai
Scientific Director and Co-Founder
Bloom IVF and BAUFICI Genetics
President, Indian Society for Assisted Reproduction (2022–2024)
President, Association of Maharashtra Obstetric and Gynaecological Societies (2020–2022)
Past President, FOGSI, IAGE, MOGS and MSR

**Nisha Bhatnagar** MBBS MD
Medical Director
Department of Reproductive Medicine
Aveya IVF Center
New Delhi, India

**Niti Vijay**
DNB (Obs and Gyne) Diploma in Clinical ART IFS
Senior Consultant and
Director of the Clinics
Department of Gynecology and IVF
Aveya Fertility, Phoenix Hospitals and The Clinics
New Delhi, India

**Pankaj Talwar** MD PhD
Director at i-Ceat | i-Consult| i-HOMaa
Dean
Department of Clinical Embryology and Reproductive Sciences
Shridhar University
Pilani, Rajasthan, India
i-HOMaa Fertility Clinic
Gurugram, Haryana, India
President, Indian Fertility Society (2024–2026)

**Pikee Saxena**
MD FICOG MNAMS FMAS FIMCH PGCC (Hospital Management) PGDCR (Clinical Research)
Director–Professor
Department of Obstetrics and Gynecology
Lady Hardinge Medical College and Associated Hospitals
New Delhi, India

**Prachi Benara**
MS DNB PG Dip (Reproductive Medicine, UK)
Senior Consultant and
Lead Clinical Trainer
Department of Reproductive Medicine
Birla Fertility and IVF
Gurugram, Haryana, India

**Pratik Tambe**
MD FICOG FICRM FICMCH FIAOG
ART Consultant
Gynec Endoscopic Surgeon
Department of Obstetrics and Gynecology, Reproductive Medicine, Gynec Endoscopic Surgery, High Risk Pregnancy
Ashirwad IVF
Mumbai, Maharashtra, India
Governing Council Member
ICOG and ICRM
Managing Committee Member
MOGS, ISAR, MSR
Past Chair, FOGSI and AMOGS Endocrinology Committees

**Rachita Munjal**
MS DAGE FRM PG Dip US
Senior Consultant and Director
Department of Fertility and IVF
Cloudnine Hospital
Gurugram, Haryana, India

**Rajapriya Ayyappan**
MD DNB MRCOG FRCOG FRM FICOG
Managing Director
Department of Obstetrics and Gynecology
Srinivas Priya Hospital and Om Fertility Center
Chennai, Tamil Nadu, India

**Renu Tanwar** DNB MNAMS
Director–Professor and IVF Coordinator
Department of Obstetrics and Gynecology
Maulana Azad Medical College
New Delhi, India

**Rishma Pai** MD FRCOG DNB FCPS FICOG
Consultant Gynecologist and Infertility Specialist
Department of Obstetrics and Gynecology, IVF
Lilavati, Jaslok, and Hinduja Hospitals
Mumbai, Maharashtra, India
Treasurer, International Federation of Fertility Societies (IFFS)
Former President, FOGSI, ISAR, IAGE
Member, FIGO Menstrual Disorders Committee

**Ruchica Goel**
DGO FICOG FICMCH FMAS DMAS
Senior Consultant IVF
Department of Obstetrics and Gynecology
Shri Ram Murti Smarak Institute of Medical Science
Bareilly, Uttar Pradesh, India

**Sarabjeet Singh**
MBBS DGO PhD Fellowship ART (1 year)
Director
Sarab Healthcare and IVF and DOVE ART Bank
Department of Reproductive Medicine and IVF
Jalandhar, Punjab, India

**Saumya Prasad** MS DMAS FMAS
Senior Consultant
Department of Obstetrics and Gynecology, IVF
Matritava Advanced IVF and Maternity Centre
New Delhi, India

**Shalu Gupta**
MS DNB MNAMS FNB (Reproductive Medicine) MRCOG (UK)
Director
Department of Reproductive Medicine and Fertility
Cloudnine Hospital
Gurugram, Haryana, India

**Shweta Mittal Gupta**
MBBS MD (Obs and Gyne) DNB
Co-Director and Senior Consultant
Centre of IVF and Human Reproduction
Sir Ganga Ram Hospital
New Delhi, India

**Siddhartha Nagireddy**
MBBS MS (Obs and Gyne) MCh (Reproductive Medicine and Surgery)
Department of Reproductive Medicine and Endoscopic Surgery
SNH Fertility and Endoscopy Center
Nellore, Andhra Pradesh, India

**Sonu Balhara** DGO DNB
Director and Senior Consultant IVF and Infertility
Department of Reproductive Medicine
ART Fertility Clinics
Gurugram, Haryana, India

**Sunita Tandulwadkar**
MD (Obs and Gyne) FICS (Gyne-Endoscopy) FICOG
President, FOGSI (2025–2026)
Gynecological Endoscopist and ART & IVF Specialist
Head, Department of Obstetrics and Gynecology
Chief, IVF & Endoscopy Center
Ruby Hall Clinic, Pune
Founder and Medical Director
Solo Clinic IVF—A Center for Excellence in Infertility and Endoscopy, Pune
Founder and Medical Director
Solo Stem Cells—A Stem Cell Research and Application Center, Pune
Founder and Director
Alive Regenerative Wellness
Pune, Maharashtra, India

**Sweta Gupta**
MD MRCOG FRCOG (UK) MSc (Bristol)
Director
Department of IVF
Max Super Speciality Hospitals
Noida, Uttar Pradesh, India

**T Chitra**
MD (Obs and Gyne) DNB MNAMS
Fellowship in RM and Laparoscopy
Professor
Department of Obstetrics and Gynecology
Jawaharlal Institute of Postgraduate Medical Education and Research
Puducherry, India

# Preface

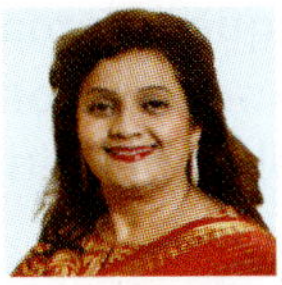

***Editor-in-Chief***
**Sunita Tandulwadkar**

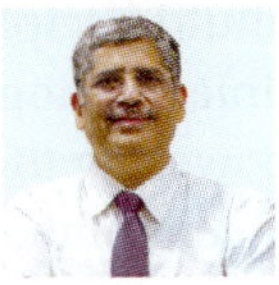

***Editor***
**Pankaj Talwar**

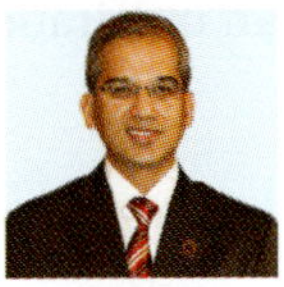

***Editor***
**Pratik Tambe**

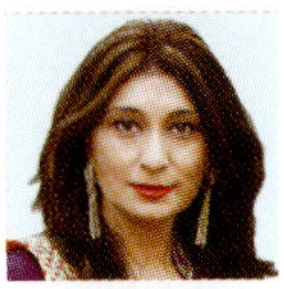

***Expert***
**Rishma Pai**

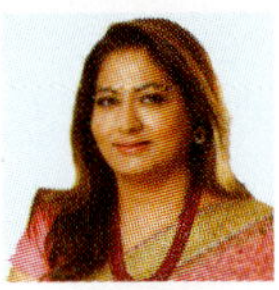

***Expert***
**Nandita Palshetkar**

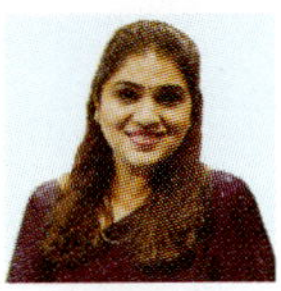

***Convener***
**Pooja Lodha**

In our pursuit of advancing women's health in India, establishing our own ethical evidence-based recommendations is essential. As the President of the Federation of Obstetric and Gynaecological Societies of India (FOGSI) 2025, I am delighted to present this *Ethical Evidence-Based Recommendations on Endometriosis*, a resource born from the dedicated efforts of experts across the country. While international bodies such as the International Federation of Gynecology and Obstetrics (FIGO), American Society for Reproductive Medicine (ASRM), ESHRE, and Royal College of Obstetricians and Gynaecologists (RCOG) have established their recommendations, India has yet to create a cohesive, evidence-backed framework. This book aims to bridge that gap, providing Indian practitioners with a comprehensive and practical set of recommendations for diagnosing and managing endometriosis.

Endometriosis, a complex condition, affects women across various life stages, each with unique manifestations and management requirements. This book begins with foundational recommendations on diagnosis, equipping practitioners with insights to accurately identify endometriosis, a vital first step toward effective care. Recognizing age-specific needs, we address the distinct presentations in adolescents and reproductive-age women, offering tailored guidance. For adolescents, early interventions are discussed, while for reproductive-age women, recommendations focus on managing endometriosis-associated pain and infertility to improve quality of life.

A major focus of this book is managing symptoms associated with endometriosis. The chapters provide recommendations for both pharmacologic and nonpharmacologic options, helping practitioners personalize care and enhance outcomes. Additionally, a dedicated section on the menopausal age group addresses special considerations for managing symptoms in older women, ensuring continuous, quality care throughout every phase of life.

The book also includes recommendations for special conditions in endometriosis, recognizing that some cases require unique approaches. These sections provide a nuanced perspective for handling complex presentations that may fall outside standard protocols, enabling practitioners to manage even challenging cases confidently.

This book represents FOGSI's commitment to equipping Indian gynecologists with the latest scientific advancements, framed within our cultural and clinical context. I am deeply grateful to the multidisciplinary team whose collaborative efforts made this publication possible. We hope this book becomes a trusted companion for practitioners, empowering them to deliver compassionate, evidence-based care for patients with endometriosis.

Through this initiative, FOGSI reaffirms its dedication to advancing women's health and setting a new standard for ethical, informed care. We trust that this book will serve as both a valuable guide and an inspiration for the management of endometriosis across India.

# Contents

CHAPTER 1

# Diagnosis of Endometriosis

*Harpreet Kaur, Maansi Jain,*
*Nisha Bhatnagar, Sweta Gupta*

## Q1. What are the common symptoms of endometriosis?

**Draft recommendation:**

- *Common symptoms of endometriosis* vary from no symptoms to debilitating pain, which may be cyclical/non-cyclical like dysmenorrhea, dyspareunia, dyschezia, pelvic pain, lower backache, infertility, heavy menstrual bleeding or atypical symptoms like irritable bowel or bladder symptoms, catamenial pneumothorax symptoms, cyclical scar swelling or pain and hematuria.
- The presence of non-specific symptoms may delay the diagnosis

**Summary of evidence:** Many women with endometriosis present with nonspecific symptoms, such as chronic lower back pain or abdominal pain, which may delay diagnosis. The presence of cyclical pain should raise a suspicion of endometriosis ESHRE endometriosis guidelines 2022. Schliep et al., 2015, ENDO study, in an operative cohort of 473 women, reported 18 unique symptoms of endometriosis with pelvic pain (92.5%), dyspareunia (80.0%), and heavy bleeding (75.0%) being the most commonly reported.

## Q2. Can diagnosis be made on symptoms alone?

**Draft recommendation**

- Endometriosis *may be* considered a probable diagnosis based on symptoms alone. The predictive value of symptoms alone for the diagnosis of endometriosis is poor except for dyschezia and severe dyspareunia, which might be predictive of endometriosis.
- Combining symptoms with USG (TVS/TRUS) and biomarkers like CA-125 and other markers statistical models may increase the predictive value.

**Summary of evidence:** Evidence to support diagnosis based on symptoms alone is weak. Severe dysmenorrhea may be predictive of endometriosis and the presence of multiple symptoms increases the chances of endometriosis. Nnoaham et al., 2012, in a large, prospective, observational, multicentric study from over 13 countries have shown a low sensitivity of the symptom-based model to predict endometriosis (sensitivity of 82.3% and specificity of 75.8%). Among all the symptoms, severe dysmenorrhea has increased predictive value of endometriosis (Hsu et al., 2010). A study on 185 women undergoing laparoscopy for chronic pelvic pain, Ballard et al., 2010, showed that throbbing pain and dyschezia could be useful for differentiating between women with endometriosis and women without endometriosis. Increasing the number of symptoms increases the predictive of endometriosis.

Research gap: In the future, well-designed randomized research studies are recommended to compare symptoms alone with various predictive models for diagnosis of endometriosis.

### Q3. Can severity of pain be correlated to the severity of the disease?

**Draft recommendation:** Severity of pain is not associated with severity of disease

**Summary of evidence:** There is no evidence to suggest that severe pain is always associated with severe disease. In a study done by Karp et al., 2023, it was found that the severity of pain seems to be independent of the endometriosis stage. Women with moderate disease may experience intense pelvic pain, while those with more severe Endometriosis may encounter less acute or chronic pain. So, endometriosis cannot be identified currently by pathogenic features or biomarkers, and the key symptoms of endometriosis like pain and infertility can mistakenly be attributed to other causes.

### Q4. Can a menstrual diary or record of symptoms be used for early diagnosis?

**Draft recommendation:**

- Keeping a symptom diary or record of symptoms may not help in early diagnosis, but it may help women identify the issues and express themselves fully
- Though currently no evidence exists that a symptom diary/questionnaire/app reduces the time to diagnosis or leads to earlier diagnosis, the ESHRE endometriosis guideline 2022 considers its potential benefit in complementing the traditional history-taking process as it aids in quantifying pain and helps women to express their symptoms.

**Summary of evidence:** In a study conducted by Kim et al., 2022, the group focused on providing consensus regarding early clinical diagnosis and they focused on symptom recognition and diagnosis without laparoscopy. For early empirical treatment, the management of women with clinical presentation suggestive of endometriosis should be individualized considering presentation and therapeutic need.

**Research gap:** Large randomized studies are needed to compare symptoms and severity of endometriosis so that a patient friendly tool is available.

### Q5. Can diagnostic methods like scan and MRI be used in endometriosis?

**Draft recommendation:** Diagnostic workup includes imaging techniques. Ultrasound (TVS/TRUS for pelvic endometriosis, TAS (extra pelvic) primarily or MRI in a few selected cases but negative findings do not exclude superficial peritoneal disease. Applying imaging methods and result interpretation can be dependent on a clinician's experience and skill (e.g., ultrasound, surgery) and the availability of the imaging equipment (e.g., MRI).

**Summary of evidence:** These have been suggestions from ESHRE endometriosis guidelines 2022.

### Q6. What is the role of laparoscopy in endometriosis?

**Draft recommendation:**

- Laparoscopy is *no longer considered a gold standard* for diagnosis of endometriosis, though it can identify superficial endometriotic spots and provide histological confirmation. Imaging combined with empirical treatment (hormonal contraceptives or progestogens) can be considered in women suspected of endometriosis. There is no evidence of superiority of either approach (laparoscopy or imaging). Pros and cons should be discussed with the patient. (ESHRE endometriosis guideline 2022)
- There is a need for adequate counselling with shared decision making for each case especially regarding ovarian reserve (reduction of antral follicle count and AMH). Clinicians should avoid surgical over correction.
- Criteria for selecting cases for laparoscopy include pain (refractory to medical management), rapid growth in the size of endometriotic cyst, suspicious features seen on ultrasound/MRI.
- Surgery for endometrioma prior to ART can be considered to improve endometriosis-associated pain or accessibility of follicles during oocyte retrieval.
- Surgical excision of deep infiltrating endometriosis (DIE) lesions prior to ART should be guided mainly by pain symptoms and patient's preference as its effectiveness on reproductive outcome is uncertain due to lack of randomized studies.

**Summary of evidence:** Zanelotti et al., 2017 discussed meta-analysis of 10 RCTs showed that Laparoscopic operative surgery was associated with decreased overall pain compared with diagnostic laparoscopy.

### Q7. How should we monitor the patients for identifying long term disease progression?

**Draft recommendation:**

- Monitoring the patients should be by history (symptoms), imaging and AMH/AFC (for those desirous of fertility).

- Follow-up and psychological support should be considered in women with confirmed endometriosis, particularly deep and ovarian endometriosis, although there is currently no evidence of benefit of regular long-term monitoring for early detection of recurrence, deep infiltrating endometriosis (DIE), or malignancy. The appropriate frequency and type of follow-up or monitoring is unknown and should be individualized based on previous and current treatments and severity of the disease and symptoms. (ESHRE endometriosis guidelines 2022).

**Summary of evidence:** Moen et al., 2022 concluded that there is little risk that asymptomatic, minimal endometriosis found incidentally will become symptomatic in a long-term follow-up study of women with asymptomatic endometriosis diagnosed incidentally at sterilization.

**Research gap:** Currently no studies of sufficient size or quality address the long-term. High-quality research is required to understand the benefits of long-term monitoring.

### Q8. How beneficial is early diagnosis in terms of preventing the course and severity of disease?

**Draft recommendation:** There is no clear-cut evidence to suggest early diagnosis to prevent severity and progression of the disease. Although adequate studies to support the benefits of early versus late diagnosis are lacking, ESHRE endometriosis guideline 2022 recommends that in symptomatic women, attempts should be made to relieve symptoms.

**Summary of evidence:** Al Shukri M et al., 2023 study was conducted to assess whether there is a specific symptom profile characteristic of endometriosis to alert physicians for earlier referrals. They concluded that no specific symptom profile appears to predict an early diagnosis of endometriosis. However, over the years the diagnosis of endometriosis is made earlier, likely due to increasing awareness of women and their physicians about the disease.

**Research gap:** High-quality research is required to evaluate the benefit of early diagnosis.

## BIBLIOGRAPHY

1. Al Shukri M, Al Riyami AS, Al Ghafri W, et al. Are There Predictors of Early Diagnosis of Endometriosis Based on Clinical Profile? A Retrospective Study. Oman Med J. 2023;38(1):e458.
2. Ballard K, Lane H, Hudelist G, et al. Can specific pain symptoms help in the diagnosis of endometriosis? A cohort study of women with chronic pelvic pain. Fertil Steril. 2010;94(1):20-7.
3. Becker CM, Bokor A, Heikinheimo O, et al. ESHRE Endometriosis Guideline Group, ESHRE guideline: endometriosis. Human Reprod Open. 2022;2:hoac009.

4. Endo Study, Schliep KC, Mumford SL, et al. Pain typology and incident endometriosis. Hum Reprod. 2015;30(10):2427-38.
5. Green IC, Burnett T, Famuyide A. Persistent pelvic pain in patients with endometriosis. Clin Obstet Gynecol. 2022;65(4):775-85.
6. Hsu AL, Khachikyan I, Stratton P. Invasive and noninvasive methods for the diagnosis of endometriosis. Clin Obstet Gynecol. 2010;53:413-9.
7. Karp BI, Stratton P. Endometriosis-associated chronic pelvic pain. Med. 2023;4:143-6.
8. Kim MR, Chapron C, Römer T, et al. Clinical Diagnosis and Early Medical Management for Endometriosis: Consensus from Asian Expert Group. Healthcare (Basel). 2022;10(12):2515.
9. Kor E, Mostafavi SRS, Mazhin ZA, et al. Relationship between the severity of endometriosis symptoms (dyspareunia, dysmenorrhea and chronic pelvic pain) and the spread of the disease on ultrasound. BMC Res Notes. 2020;13(1):546.
10. Martire FG, Lazzeri L, Conway F, et al. Adolescence and endometriosis: symptoms, ultrasound signs and early diagnosis. Fertil Steril. 2020;114(5):1049-57.
11. Martire FG, Russo C, Selntigia A, et al. Early noninvasive diagnosis of endometriosis: dysmenorrhea and specific ultrasound findings are important indicators in young women. Fertil Steril. 2023;119(3):455-464.
12. Moen MH, Stokstad T. A long-term follow-up study of women with asymptomatic endometriosis diagnosed incidentally at sterilization. Fertil Steril. 2022;78:4:773-6.
13. Nnoaham KE, Hummelshoj L, Kennedy SH, et al. World Endometriosis Research Foundation Women's Health Symptom Survey Consortium Developing symptom-based predictive models of endometriosis as a clinical screening tool: results from a multicenter study. Fertil Steril. 2012;98(3):692-701.e5.
14. Spirit Hunsche E, Gauthier M, Witherspoon B, et al. Endometriosis Symptoms and Their Impacts on the Daily Lives of US Women: Results from an Interview Study. Int J Womens Health. 2023;15:893-904.
15. Zanelotti A, Decherney AH. Surgery and Endometriosis. Clin Obstet Gynecol. 2017;60(3):477-84.

CHAPTER 2

# Endometriosis in Adolescent Age Group

*Sarabjeet Singh, Saumya Prasad,*
*Siddhartha Nagireddy, Shweta Mittal Gupta*

## Q1. How to diagnose and manage endometriosis in adolescents?

**Draft recommendation:**

- Conduct a thorough medical history and clinical evaluation, focusing on age at menarche, menstrual characteristics, medication use, family history of endometriosis, and related symptoms such as gastrointestinal issues, nausea, and fatigue (RCOG, Green-top Guidelines No. 41; 2012).
- Utilize ultrasound (preferably transabdominal or transrectal in pre-sexually active adolescents) and MRI for imaging. MRI is particularly recommended when ultrasound results are inconclusive or transrectal evaluation is not acceptable.
- Avoid surgical confirmation of endometriosis in adolescents. Instead, follow non-invasive diagnostic pathways based on ESHRE endometriosis guidelines.
- Tailor treatment based on the patient's symptoms, side effect tolerance, and progression of the disease.
- Use hormonal contraceptives or progestins (such as Dienogest) as first-line treatment for adolescents with endometriosis-related pain. Continuous oral contraceptive therapy is more effective than cyclic therapy for managing dysmenorrhea (Sasamoto N et al.).
- For adolescents intolerant to oral medication, consider subcutaneous implants like etonogestrel (ENG) or an LNG-IUS device with appropriate counselling. GnRH agonists can be used as second-line therapy, with add-back therapy to prevent side effects like bone loss.
- Reserve surgery for cases with specific conditions such as rapidly growing ovarian cysts, suspicion of malignancy or persistent pain unresponsive to medical treatment. (Janssen EB et al., 2013). During surgery, focus on preserving fertility and minimizing damage to healthy tissues using techniques like stripping and $CO_2$ laser vaporization.
- Patients should be counselled appropriately for oocyte freezing preferably before they reach the age of 35 years to significantly increase their chances of success (Cobo A et al., 2021) or ovarian tissue cryopreservation.

**Summary of evidence:** *ESHRE* endometriosis guideline 2022 (Becker CM; Bokor A et al., 2022) guidelines proposes a careful history to identify possible risk factors for endometriosis must be taken which includes a positive family history, obstructive genital malformations, early menarche, or short menstrual cycle.

Transvaginal ultrasound is recommended to be used in adolescents in whom it is appropriate, as it is effective in diagnosing ovarian endometriosis. If the scan is not appropriate, MRI, transabdominal, trans-perineal, or transrectal scan may be considered.

ESHRE 2022 guidelines also recommend hormonal contraceptives or progestogens (systemically or via LNG-IUS) should be prescribed as the first line hormonal therapy because they may be effective and safe. However, it is important to note that some progestogens may decrease bone mineral density.

**Evidence gap:** There is a need for more accurate, non-invasive biomarkers for diagnosing endometriosis in adolescents. Current biomarkers, such as CA-125, lack specificity, highlighting the need for further research into the inflammatory and autoimmune aspects of endometriosis to develop more reliable diagnostic tools (Becker et al., 2022).

There is a lack of consensus on the most effective hormonal therapy for different age groups and patient types, particularly in adolescents.

Further research is needed to evaluate the long-term effects of progestins and continuous hormonal therapy on future fertility.

## BIBLIOGRAPHY

1. Becker CM, Bokor A, Heikinheimo O, et al. ESHRE guideline: endometriosis. Hum Reprod Open. 2022;2022(2): hoac009.
2. Cobo A, García-Velasco JA, Remohí J, et al. Oocyte vitrification for fertility preservation for both medical and nonmedical reasons. Fertil Steril. 2021;115(5):1091-1101.
3. Janssen EB, Rijkers AC, Hoppenbrouwers K, et al. Prevalence of endometriosis diagnosed by laparoscopy in adolescents with dysmenorrhea or chronic pelvic pain: a systematic review. Hum Reprod Update. 2013;19:570-82.
4. RCOG Green top guideline No 41, 2012
5. Sasamoto N, DePari M, Vitonis AF, et al. Evaluation of CA125 in relation to pain symptoms among adolescents and young adult women with and without surgically-confirmed endometriosis. PLoS One. 2020;15(8):e0238043.

CHAPTER 3

# Endometriosis in Reproductive Age Group

## 3.1 TREATMENT OF ENDOMETRIOSIS ASSOCIATED PAIN

*T Chitra, Pikee Saxena, Ruchica Goel*

### Q1. Can analgesic effectively control symptoms in endometriosis (EAPP)?

**Draft recommendations:**

- NSAIDs or other analgesics either alone or in combination may be offered to women with other treatments to reduce endometriosis-associated pelvic pain (EAPP).
- All the options are equally effective. No analgesic has been found to be superior to the others as per the available evidence.

**Summary of evidence:** Medical treatment of suspected or confirmed EAPP is initially by the use of over-the-counter, simple analgesics like paracetamol and non-steroidal anti-inflammatory drugs (NSAIDs).

Neuromodulators (e.g., antidepressants, selective serotonin uptake inhibitors or anticonvulsants) are recommended for the management of chronic or persistent pain. Neuromodulators differ from conventional analgesics, such as NSAIDs, in that they primarily affect the central nervous system's modulation of pain rather than peripheral mediators of inflammation.).

Emerging evidence suggests that cabergoline, a vascular endothelial growth factor pathway inhibitor, is an effective therapeutic option for women with EAPP, Divasta et al., 2021.

Analgesics may be used in combination with surgery and/or hormonal treatments. However, analgesics may cause gastrointestinal adverse effects and do not prevent disease progression.

### Q2. Are hormonal therapies effective in pain control in endometriosis (EAPP)?

**Draft recommendations:**

- Clinicians should encourage *shared decision-making* after thorough counselling about risks and benefits including adverse effects, efficacy, costs, patient's preferences and availability into consideration when choosing hormone treatments for EAPP.

- *Routes of hormonal treatment* can be oral, vaginal, transdermal, intrauterine. However, oral and intrauterine is preferred in our country by health care providers.
- *Therapeutic Options available to health care providers are* combined hormonal pill, progesterone only pills, GnRH agonists, GnRH antagonist or Aromatase inhibitors. (Alonso et al., 2024).
- *Lines of management*

  First line:
  - Oral options are combined hormonal contraceptive pills (OCP) or progestogens.
  - Oral combined hormonal contraceptives ( progestin synthetic form of the hormone progestogen/progesterone) and estrogen (usually ethinyl estradiol or 17β estradiol) usually continuously from 3 to 6 months to reduce endometriosis associated dyspareunia, dysmenorrhea and non-menstrual pain. As OCP is cost effective (cheap), considered safe and often required for contraception.
  - *Oral progestogens* can be dydrogesterone, 10 mg thrice daily continuously is helpful as immunomodulator especially in women desirous of fertility. Dienogest, 2 mg/day continuously can be used continuously up to 52 weeks (Muzii et al., 2022).
  - *Combined oral contraceptive pills* containing ethynyl estradiol and Dienogest 2 mg can be considered in Indian context due to similar efficacy and better cost effectiveness as mono therapy (Cho et al., 2022).
  - *Levonorgestrel-releasing intrauterine system* or an etonogestrel releasing subdermal implant can be offered to reduce EAPP. Levonorgestrel-releasing intrauterine system (LNG-IUS, 20 microgram/day) can be kept up to 7 years

  Second line: *GnRH agonists and GnRH antagonists* can be offered as *second line* if hormonal contraceptives or progestogen are ineffective to reduce EAPP due to their side effects. Along with GnRH, combined hormonal add-back therapy should be added to prevent bone loss and hypoestrogenic symptoms.

  Third line: *Aromatase inhibitors* are recommended in women with *refractory* endometriosis-associated pain not responding to other medical or surgical treatment. They can be prescribed in combination with other hormonal therapy.

**Summary of evidence:** Rationale for treating endometriosis associated pain with hormonal contraceptives is that they modify the hormonal milieu either by suppressing ovarian activity or acting directly on steroid receptors and enzymes found in the lesions.

All hormonal treatments reduce EAPP as compared to placebo (National Institute for Health and Care Excellence, 2017). Magnitude of hormonal treatment effect has been shown to be similar for all treatments indicating that there is little difference between their capacity to reduce pain and none of these therapies are free of side effects. In clinical practice, the efficacy and side-effect profiles of these therapies are highly individualized.

Contraceptive properties of the hormones are not desirable for women seeking fertility treatment but may be useful if the woman does not wish to become pregnant.

### Q3. How effective is surgery for pain relief in endometriosis?

**Draft recommendations:**

- Available routes are open, laparoscopy, and robotic-assisted laparoscopy. Laparoscopic surgery is preferred over the robotic route as it does not offer significant advantage over conventional in terms of clinical outcome (Song et al.).
- Laparoscopic adhesiolysis, excision, coagulation and laser vaporization of endometriotic tissue are the different techniques available.

*Superficial endometriosis*

- *Excision* is preferred over ablation for patients with moderate to severe superficial endometriosis and those with deep infiltrating lesions. Excision is recommended to reduce endometriosis-associated pain refractory to medical and hormonal treatment in cases where fertility is not desired.

*Pelvic adhesions*

- Adhesiolysis is performed to restore anatomy of the pelvis.

*Endometrioma*

- Laparoscopically excision (*cystectomy*) is preferred over ablation.

*Deep infiltrating endometriosis*

- For patients with deep infiltrating endometriosis (DIE), surgical intervention (excision) should be comprehensive, with a multidisciplinary approach when necessary (involving colorectal or urological surgeons).
- Combine surgery with postoperative hormonal (progesterone) management for optimal long-term pain relief and to reduce recurrence rates
- Patients should be counselled about the possibility of recurrence and the need for ongoing management.

**Summary of evidence:** Laparoscopic surgery should be preferred over laparotomy, especially for severe endometriosis because of less pain, shorter duration of hospitalization, quicker recovery and better cosmetic result. A meta-analysis by Restaino S et al., in 2020 of the available studies, showed no other difference in perioperative outcomes between robotic and conventional laparoscopic surgery, except the longer time that is needed in robotic surgery. A meta-analysis by Pundir J et al., in 2017 of randomized controlled trials, involving 335 women found that excision of endometriosis was more effective than coagulation in reducing dysmenorrhea, dyschezia, and chronic pelvic pain at a 12-month follow-up.

ESHRE endometriosis guideline 2022 emphasized that surgical treatment of endometriomas, whether by cystectomy or ablation, can diminish ovarian reserve and negatively impact fertility. This risk is heightened for women with large, recurrent, or bilateral endometriomas and it is advisable to measure AMH levels before undergoing ovarian surgery.

Surgical management of endometriotic lesions can offer a potential cure with improvements in pain and quality of life while avoiding long-term medical treatment side effects. Evidence suggests that surgical treatment for deep dyspareunia results in better outcomes and fewer side effects compared to medical treatment. However, the potential complications of extensive surgery must always be thoroughly discussed with the patient beforehand.

DIE can distort the anatomy, leading to indistinct planes of dissection. Surgery in these patients can be challenging due to high vascularity and invasive nature and may lead to even more devastating effects. The surgeon must be comfortable dissecting the retroperitoneal spaces for optimal dissection of DIE.

All guidelines, except those of NICE and ASRM, recommend excising deep infiltrating endometriosis nodules for pain associated with endometriosis. ESHRE notes that surgery in women with deep endometriosis is linked to significant intraoperative and postoperative complication rates (Kalaitzopoulos DR et al., 2021). These patients need to be informed regarding potential risks, benefits, and long-term effects on quality of life.

Surgical nerve interruption techniques like laparoscopic uterine nerve ablation (LUNA) and laparoscopic presacral neurectomy (LPSN), when combined with surgical resection, have limited supporting evidence.

Patients who do not respond to conservative treatment and are not willing for conception can be offered hysterectomy with or without removal of ovaries with excision of all visible endometriotic deposits.

### Q4. Is complementary/alternative therapy effective in relieving endometriosis associated pelvic pain (EAPP)?

**Draft recommendation:**

- EAPP has a significant adverse impact on quality of life (QoL)
- Medical and surgical treatment are associated with various side effects and risk of recurrence.
- Self-management therapies help patients to have control over pain when living with chronic debilitating conditions.
- Complimentary or alternative medical (CAM) therapies may help to reduce pain and improve quality of life. The various options for

non-medical or complementary alternative medicine (CAM) include acupuncture, electrotherapy (TENS), physiotherapy and exercise including yoga, herbal medicine, and nutritional therapy.
- CAM is associated with potential benefits and any significant harm is unclear.

**Summary of evidence:** Endometriosis is a condition associated with chronic pelvic pain. Painful symptoms are also associated with psychological stress, low self-esteem, and depression impairing physical, mental, and social well-being and reducing quality of life (QoL).

There is an increasing interest in self-management therapies so patient have control on pain when living with chronic debilitating condition.

The various options for non-medical or complementary alternative medicine (CAM) include acupuncture, electrotherapy (TENS), physiotherapy and exercise including yoga, herbal medicine, and nutritional therapy.

*Acupuncture:* Giese N et al., in 2023 published a systematic review and meta-analysis on acupuncture for endometriosis which included six studies with a total 331 patients. They found evidence for benefit for acupuncture on overall pelvic pain, menstrual pain and non-specified pelvic pain. The possible mechanisms of action include: a decrease in prostaglandin levels, decreases in nerve growth factor, increases in endogenous opioid release, and a decrease in mechanical allodynia. Most studies reported low rates of adverse events.

*Transcutaneous electrical neurostimulation:* Transcutaneous electrical neurostimulation (TENS) is based on the principle that it releases natural painkillers called endorphins from the body. Very limited data is available on the role of electrotherapy in endometriosis as no meta-analysis is available.

*Physiotherapy, behavioral therapy, and yoga:* These are known to reduce inflammation, alleviating pain and so improving quality of life. A systematic review by Tennfjord MK et al., in 2021, on the effect of physical activity and exercise on endometriosis-associated symptoms included 3 studies. Only one study found improvements in pain intensity. A quantitative meta-analysis could not be performed as the study lacked uniformity in outcomes and had several confounding factors.

*Chinese herbal medicine:* Effect of Chinese herbal medicine (CHM) on EAPP has been studied in various studies with varying results. A meta-analysis aimed to provide evidence for the efficacy and safety of CHM for EAPP had a statistically significant pooled benefit on dysmenorrhoea at the end of 3-month treatment which persisted for 3 months post treatment. It appears to have benefits in relieving EAPP with fewer side effects than traditional treatment.

*Diet:* Diet can play an important role as a modifiable risk factor affecting severity and progression of endometriosis. Nutrients have direct or indirect anti-inflammatory properties which might influence endometriosis-related pain, but evidence is not yet available for development of a specific endometriosis diet.

**Research gap:**

- There is a lack of robust studies specifically addressing the role of non-medical therapies for treatment of endometriosis related pain.
- Adequately designed trials are needed to define the potential benefits of non-medical interventions (nutrition, Chinese medicine, electrotherapy, acupuncture, physiotherapy, exercise, and psychological interventions) in endometriosis.

## 3.2 TREATMENT OF ENDOMETRIOSIS-ASSOCIATED INFERTILITY

*Bindu Bajaj, Rajapriya Ayyappan, Pankaj Talwar*

### Q1. Does medical treatment enhance fertility in endometriosis?

**Draft recommendations:**

- Medical treatment does not enhance fertility in Endometriosis.
- There is insufficient evidence that administration of GnRH agonist therapy or hormonal therapies prior to ART increases live birth rates. There is insufficient evidence to recommend aromatase inhibitors, COC, Progesterone as pre-treatment prior to ART to increase live birth rates.

**Summary of evidence:** The role of medical therapy in infertility associated with endometriosis is mainly to neutralize the proinflammatory cytokines so as to prevent oxidative stress. This may improve oocyte quality and increase the pregnancy rates.

Continuous GnRH agonist (GnRH-a) administration for a period of 3 to 6 months causes a down-regulation of GnRH-a receptors on pituitary gland and a severe hypo-estrogenic state, causing suppression of endometriotic lesions. Ovulation stimulation thereafter was earlier thought to increase pregnancy rates in ART cycles. However, systematic reviews have shown conflicting evidence and the potential need for higher doses of gonadotropins.

Orally active aromatase inhibitors (AIs) have gained attention for treatment of infertile women with endometriosis in whom aromatase p450 is aberrantly expressed.

### Q2. Can surgical treatment enhance fertility in endometriosis?

**Draft recommendations:**

- Laparoscopic ablation of endometrial implants in infertile women may increase pregnancy rates if performed. However, diagnostic laparoscopy is no longer considered standard care for endometriosis.

- Ovarian cystectomy for an endometrioma is indicated to relieve pain and increase accessibility of follicles during OPU in ART cycles. However, surgery may result in depletion of AFC and reduction of AMH.
- Ovarian endometriotic cyst aspiration should not be performed as it may recur and the ovary is prone to infections and abscess formation. If inadvertently puncture happens during OPU, broad-spectrum antibiotics should be given and close post-operative monitoring should be done.
- Endometriosis Fertility Index (EFI) may be used to identify and counsel patients who will be benefited with ART, as it is a validated, reproducible and cost-effective tool.

**Summary of evidence:** The objective of surgical treatment for endometriosis is to restore anatomic relationship and to ablate visible endometriotic lesions.

*Ablation of endometriosis implants:* Ablation of peritoneal implants may be done electrosurgical or by excision. Bafort et al., 2020-cochrane review concluded that laparoscopic surgery increases viable intrauterine pregnancy rates compared to diagnostic laparoscopy only. The study included 14 RCTs and compared the effectiveness and safety of laparoscopic surgery with other laparoscopic or robotic intervention, medical treatment, or diagnostic laparoscopy only.

Meta-analysis by Hodgson, et al., 2020 found that infertile women with surgically confirmed endometriosis benefitted from surgical laparoscopy alone. However, similar to other RCTs, in this analysis the live births and miscarriages were poorly reported in outcomes.

*Endometrioma excision:* Incidence of ovarian endometriomas in women with endometriosis is 17–44%. These are associated with a more advanced stage of disease (ASRM stages III and IV). Endometrioma cyst wall excision improves the rate of spontaneous pregnancy in sub fertile individuals but has no impact when advanced reproductive technologies such as in vitro fertilization (IVF) are employed. Presence of ovarian endometriomas during ART cycles may cause difficulty in oocyte retrieval thereby necessitating their surgical removal. Endometrioma resection has not been shown to improve IVF/intracytoplasmic sperm injection (ICSI) outcomes and therefore is not advised for this indication.

Alborzi S et al., 2019 have shown that the rate of endometrioma recurrence after laparoscopic ovarian cystectomy is 6–67%, while the rate of recurrence after aspiration is 28–98%. In addition, when compared to fulguration or coagulation, pregnancy rates were found to be higher in patients that underwent cystectomy. They reported pregnancy rates that were similar after laparoscopic stripping technique (72.2%) or cyst vaporization with $CO_2$ fiber laser (74.3%). However, spontaneous pregnancy rate was higher after laparoscopic stripping (55.5% vs. 35.9%).

*Endometriosis Fertility Index (EFI)* was developed as an end-of-surgery scoring system that predicts non-ART pregnancy rates (natural conception or IUI) after surgery. It was derived from prospective analysis of clinical data and has since been (externally) validated in over 30 studies, of which the majority were evaluated in a meta-analysis (Vesali et al., 2020). Confirming its good performance despite substantial heterogeneity between studies. By scoring patient-related factors (age, duration of subfertility and history of prior pregnancy) and surgical factors ("least function score" of the tubes and ovaries, endometriosis lesion and total score as extracted from the rASRM staging) factors, a score between 0 and 10 is generated. This score is strongly correlated with postoperative non-ART pregnancy rates and can therefore be used to counsel patients on their reproductive options, although it assumes normal gamete function.

### Q3. What is the role of ART in endometriosis?

**Draft recommendation:**

- There is sufficient evidence to support the use of ART to enhance fertility. The modalities of treatment may vary from intrauterine insemination (IUI) to IVF depending upon the age of the patient, AFC, AMH and tubal patency. Even the stage 3 and 4 endometriosis patients may benefit from Controlled ovarian stimulation and IUI.
- For advanced stages of endometriosis with increasing age with low ovarian reserve, IVF is the preferred modality.
- All controlled ovarian hyper stimulation (COH) protocols are equally effective though the dose of gonadotropins may increase with use of an agonist cycle.
- The quality of oocytes, embryos, and live birth rates in ART with endometriosis were similar to non-endometriosis in IVF.
- ART is safe in endometriosis though we need to avoid OHSS and avoid inadvertent injury to endometrioma leading to pelvic infections.
- A new marker BCL 6 for endometrial receptivity has been recently used. A high level is associated with adverse IVF outcomes.

**Summary of evidence:** Alshehre et al., 2021 in a systematic review analysis in women with endometrioma versus controls, total number of mature oocytes retrieved, total number of embryos, implantation rates, clinical pregnancy and live births were similar.

Impact of ART on endometriosis-ART does not increase the recurrence of endometriosis. It also has no effect on birth outcomes of patients conceived following ART in endometriosis

A new marker for endometrial receptivity in endometriosis emerged: BCL 6, a biomarker for endometrial inflammation as it stimulates endometrial cytokine expression. Prospective cohort data provide a proof of concept that high BCL 6 expression is associated with adverse IVF outcomes in women with endometriosis and that patients with high BCL 6 expression may benefit from medical and surgical treatment prior to IVF (Miijatovic et al., 2024).

Currently there is uncertainty as to whether long-term GnRH agonist therapy is beneficial when compared to standard IVF/ICSI in endometriosis. In addition, there is no evidence to support the use of oral GnRH antagonists and oral contraceptives as pre-treatment prior to ART, but results of ongoing studies will determine further (Miijatovic et al., 2024).

### Q4. What is the role of fertility preservation in endometriosis?

**Draft recommendation:**

- Elective egg freezing (EEF) is safe and standard fertility preservation treatment preferably before 35 years. It can be recommended to women affected by endometriosis when they decide to postpone motherhood due to career, education or lack of suitable partner, as the disease leads to subfertility and poor oocyte quality. However, low-return usage rates, low cost-effectiveness, elicits controversy, medical and ethical concerns.
- Ovarian tissue cryopreservation may be discussed though the benefit remains unknown.

**Summary of evidence:** According to Richard et al., 2020 fertility preservation in patients of endometriosis should be considered in selected patients taking into consideration age, risk of ovarian damage, those with bilateral ovarian endometriomas or those with unilaterally operated endometrioma with a contralateral recurrence.

Ideally, oocyte preservation should be done before 35 years of age.

Ovarian reserve testing and appropriate counselling can help to counsel women in egg freezing for endometriosis affected women seeking future fertility. Unreasonable postponing of pregnancy must not be encouraged.

## BIBLIOGRAPHY

1. Alborzi S, Zahiri Sorouri Z, Askari E, et al. The success of various endometrioma treatments in infertility: a systematic review and meta-analysis of prospective studies. Reprod Med Biol. 2019;18(4):312-22.
2. Alonso A, Gunther K, Maheux-Lacroix S, et al. Medical management of endometriosis. Curr Opin Obstet Gynecol. 2024;36(5):353-61.
3. Alshehre SM, Narice BF, Fenwick MA, et al. The impact of endometrioma on in vitro fertilization/intracytoplasmic injection IVF/ICSI reproductive outcomes: a systematic review and meta-analysis. Arch Gynecol Obstet. 2021;303(1):3-16.
4. Bafort C, Beebeejaun Y, Tomassetti C, et al. Laparoscopic surgery for endometriosis. Cochrane Database Syst Rev. 2020;10(10):CD011031.
5. Becker CM, Bokor A, Heikinheimo O, et al. ESHRE Endometriosis Guideline Group, ESHRE guideline: endometriosis. Hum Reprod Open. 2022 Feb 26; 2022(2):hoac009.
6. Brown J, Crawford TJ, Allen C, et al. Nonsteroidal anti-inflammatory drugs for pain in women with endometriosis. Cochrane Database Syst Rev. 2017;1:Cd004753.
7. Cho B, Roh JW, Park J, et al. Safety and Effectiveness of Dienogest (Visanne®) for Treatment of Endometriosis: A Large Prospective Cohort Study. Reprod Sci. 2020;27(3):905-15.

8. DiVasta AD, Stamoulis C, Gallagher JS, et al. Nonhormonal therapy for endometriosis: a randomized, placebo-controlled, pilot study of cabergoline versus norethindrone acetate. F S Rep. 2021;2(4):454-61.
9. Donnez J, Taylor HS, Taylor RN, et al. Treatment of endometriosis-associated pain with linzagolix, an oral gonadotropin-releasing hormone-antagonist: a randomized clinical trial. Fertil Steril. 2020;114(1):44-55.
10. ESHRE Guideline Group on Female Fertility Preservation; Anderson RA, Amant F, et al. ESHRE guideline: female fertility preservation. Human Reprod Open. 2020;4:hoaa052.
11. Giese N, Kwon KK, Armour M. Acupuncture for endometriosis: a systematic review and meta-analysis. Integr Med Res. 2023;12(4):101003.
12. Grandi G, Barra F, Ferrero S, et al. Hormonal contraception in women with endometriosis: a systematic review. Eur J Contracept Reprod Health Care. 2019;24:61-70.
13. Hodgson RM, Lee HL, Wang R, et al. Interventions for endometriosis-related infertility: a systematic review and network meta-analysis. Fertil Steril. 2020;113:374-82.e3720.
14. Horne AW, Vincent K, Hewitt CA, et al. Gabapentin for chronic pelvic pain in women (GaPP2): a multicentre, randomised, double-blind, placebo-controlled trial. Lancet. 2020;396:909-17.
15. Kalaitzopoulos DR, Samartzis N, Kolovos GN, et al. Treatment of endometriosis: a review with comparison of 8 guidelines. BMC Womens Health. 2021;21:397.
16. Mijatovic V. O-056 Can we tailor ART to endometriosis patients? Human Reprod. 2024;39.
17. Muzii L, Di Tucci C, Galati G, et al. The efficacy of dienogest in reducing disease and pain recurrence after endometriosis surgery: a systematic review and meta-analysis. Reprod Sci. 2023;30(11):3135-43.
18. Pundir J, Omanwa K, Kovoor E, et al. Laparoscopic excision versus ablation for endometriosis-associated pain: an updated systematic review and meta-analysis. J Minim Invasive Gynecol. 2017;24:747-56.
19. Restaino S, Mereu L, Finelli A, et al. Robotic surgery vs laparoscopic surgery in patients with diagnosis of endometriosis: a systematic review and meta-analysis. J Robot Surg. 2020;14(5):687-94.
20. Skorupskaite K, Hardy M, Bhandari H, et al. Evidence Based Management of Patients with Endometriosis Undergoing Assisted Conception: British Fertility Society Policy and Practice Recommendations. Human Fertil. 2024;27(1).
21. Song Z, Li S, Luo M, et al. Assessing the role of robotic surgery versus laparoscopic surgery in patients with a diagnosis of endometriosis: a meta-analysis. Medicine (Baltimore). 2023;102(50):e33104.
22. Tang H, Wu R, Li X, et al. Curative effect of 1.88-mg and 3.75-mg gonadotropin-releasing hormone agonist on stage III-IV endometriosis: randomized controlled study. J Obstet Gynaecol. 2017;43:1550-4.
23. Tennfjord MK, Gabrielsen R, Tellum T. Effect of physical activity and exercise on endometriosis-associated symptoms: a systematic review. BMC Womens Health. 2021;21(1):355.
24. Vesali S, Razavi M, Rezaeinejad M, et al. Endometriosis fertility index for predicting non-assisted reproductive technology pregnancy after endometriosis surgery: a systematic review and metaanalysis. Bjog. 2020;127:800-09.

CHAPTER 4

# Endometriosis in Menopausal Age Group

*Niti Vijay*

## Q1. How to manage endometriosis in menopause?

**Draft recommendation:**

- There can be a recurrence of endometriosis after menopause. Transformation of endometriotic lesions into malignant lesions rarely can occur, although the incidence is low.
- Menopausal Hormone Replacement (MHT) can be offered cautiously after considering patient age, severity, residual disease, comorbidities, BMI and family history after both natural and surgical menopause
- Combined MHT with estrogen and progesterone should be preferred. Estrogen only MHT should not be given. Non-hormonal MHT (e.g., Tibolone) can be considered with regular monitoring at regular intervals.
- Patients should be advised to report immediately if they have any pain or urinary or bowel symptoms. MHT should be stopped if recurrence is ascertained. A biopsy of the lesions should be taken to rule out malignancy. If a pelvic mass is detected, the work-up and treatment should be performed according to national oncology guidelines.
- Aromatase inhibitors can be given if surgery is contraindicated.

**Summary of evidence:** Several case reports and series have highlighted the potential recurrence of endometriosis and malignant transformation of the lesions in postmenopausal women due to exogenous estrogen given in the form of MHT (Gemmell et al., 2017; Sjögren et al., 2016).

*MHT with combined estrogen and progesterone:* However, the benefits of combined MHT in postmenopausal women must be considered. The key lies in selecting the correct type of MHT and the right dose at the right time. (ESHRE endometriosis guideline 2022). However, the evidence is limited. Endometriosis in postmenopausal women can also occur in the absence of MHT, which could be due to recurrence or, de novo, generation of new lesions.

*Non-hormonal:* There can also be *non-hormonal management options,* like Tibolone, a synthetic steroid with estrogenic, progestogenic, and androgenic effects. Other non-hormonal options include selective estrogen receptor modulators (SERMs) like Raloxifene, which can provide some of the benefits of estrogen without the risks (Gemmell et al., 2017).

*Recurrence of endometriosis* after MHT can be managed surgically or medically. Surgical treatment with appropriate biopsy of the lesions to rule out malignancy is essential (Streuli et al., 2017, ESHRE 2022).

*If surgery is contraindicated,* aromatase inhibitors can be used for symptomatic treatment. (ESHRE 2022, Polyzos et al., 2011)

**Research gap:** Large randomized trials and adequately powered observational studies are crucial to answer the questions on types of MHT, timings and duration in patients with menopause and a history of endometriosis.

## BIBLIOGRAPHY

1. Becker CM, Bokor A, Heikinheimo O, et al. ESHRE guideline: endometriosis. Hum Reprod Open. 2022;2022(2):hoac009.
2. Bendon CL, Becker CM. Potential mechanisms of postmenopausal endometriosis. Maturitas. 2012;72:214-19.
3. Bulun SE, Yang S, Fang Z, et al. Estrogen production and metabolism in endometriosis. Ann NY Acad Sci. 2002;955:75-85.
4. Gemmell LC, Webster KE, Kirtley S, et al. The management of menopause in women with a history of endometriosis: a systematic review. Hum Reprod Update. 2017;23:481-500.
5. Giarenis I, Giamougiannis P, Speakman CT, et al. Recurrent endometriosis following total hysterectomy with oophorectomy mimicking a malignant neoplastic lesion: a diagnostic and therapeutic challenge. Arch Gynecol Obstet. 2009;279:419-21.
6. Hickman TN, Namnoum AB, Hinton EL, et al. Timing of estrogen replacement therapy following hysterectomy with oophorectomy for endometriosis. Obstet Gynecol. 1998;91:6.
7. Polyzos NP, Fatemi HM, Zavos A, et al. Aromatase inhibitors in postmenopausal endometriosis. Reprod Biol Endocrinol. 2011;9:90.
8. Rattanachaiyanont M, Tanmahasamut P, Angsuwatthana S, et al. Hormonal replacement therapy in surgical menopause with underlying endometriosis. J Med Assoc Thai. 2003;86:702-7.
9. Sjogren LL, Morch LS, Lokkegaard E. Hormone replacement therapy and the risk of endometrial cancer: a systematic review. Maturitas. 2016;91:25-35.
10. Streuli I, Gaitzsch H, Wenger J-M, et al. Endometriosis after menopause: Physiopathology and management of an uncommon condition. Climacteric. 2017;20:138-43.

CHAPTER 5

# Special Conditions in Endometriosis

*Sarabjeet Singh, Saumya Prasad, Sonu Balhara, Prachi Banera, Rachita Munjal, Renu Tanwar, Shalu Gupta*

## Q1. How can we prevent and manage recurrence of endometriosis?

**Draft recommendations:**

- Endometriosis recurrence should be managed with a combination of surgical and medical strategies. Complete cystectomy with minimal damage to ovarian stroma is preferred to reduce recurrence risk.
- Postoperative long-term hormonal therapy, such as LNG-IUS or oral contraceptives, Dienogest is recommended to further prevent recurrence.
- Sclerotherapy may be considered by instilling alcoholic substances inside the cyst to destroy the pseudocapsule of the endometrioma.

**Summary of evidence:** Recurrence in endometriosis can be very frustrating for both patients as well as treating physicians. Lee N, et al., 2020 reported that recurrence incidence varies from very low (0%) to very high (almost 100%) in some cases. The difference in the quoted recurrence rate in the literature is attributed to various factors like a lack of appropriate definition of recurrence, difference in the pre and post-operative usage of medical treatment, difference in the study designs, stage of disease, type of surgery, skill of surgeon and deficiency of uniformity in the criteria to diagnose the recurrence. Muzii et al. (2021) concluded that when surgery is indicated, the stripping technique should still be considered as the procedure of choice, since it is associated with lower recurrence rates compared to ablative techniques.

ESHRE Endometriosis guideline development group 2022 has defined recurrence with four types of diagnostic modalities.

1. Symptom based suspected recurrence e.g. pain in the form of dyspareunia, dysmenorrhea or pelvic pain, but not proven/confirmed by imaging or surgery
2. Imaging based suspected recurrence: Like an ultrasound confirming endometrioma
3. Laparoscopically proven recurrence in the form of visible lesions but not proved by histopathology.
4. Histologically proven recurrence: Proved by histopathology during Surgery

Li XY, et al., 2019 described the risk factors which are associated with increased chances of endometriosis recurrence as:

- *Type of surgery:* A cystectomy instead of drainage and electrocoagulation has lesser chances of recurrence
- A large endometrioma (>4 cm) or advanced disease has more chances of postoperative recurrence
- Severe clinical symptoms like dysmenorrhea
- Pre or postoperative usage of medical treatment as suppressed endometriosis may recur
- Patient-related factors like positive family history or lower age at surgery
- Presence of adenomyosis.

Secondary prevention of endometriosis recurrence is aimed at keeping the resurgence of the disease to minimum (if not completely halted).

*Ovarian cystectomy with complete cyst wall removal:* Becker CM, et al., 2022 quoted that cyst wall removal without damaging the stroma by overdoing the surgery or electrocautery provides the greatest chance to remove the disease and chances of recurrence are lesser as compared to simple drainage and coagulation. However, the impact of the surgery on Ovarian reserve should be discussed with the couple which tends to get low after surgery.

**Postoperative medical treatment:** Options are combined oral contraceptive pills, LNG-IUS, progesterones.

A long term (>6 months) of postoperative medical treatment can decrease the chances of recurrence. In this context, A two-year (18–24 months) usage of a levonorgestrel-releasing intrauterine system (52 mg LNG-IUS) or a combined hormonal oral contraceptive pill (Cyclical or continuous, depending upon the patient's preference) significantly decreases the chances of endometriosis recurrence after the surgery.

A similar effectiveness was noted by Peng C, et al., 2021 with the usage of other progesterones like dydrogesterone, nor-ethisterone or dienogest. Although not recommended to be used for longer duration, Surrey ES, et al., 2022 specified that GnRH agonist if used for 6 months alone or 12 months with co-administration of OCP also decreases the chances of endometriosis recurrence.

During the ART treatment, the associated increase in the hormones particularly estrogen has been linked with the increase in chance of endometriosis recurrence and ART outcome. But data from the recent studies from Asadzadeh N, et al., 2021 refutes any association of endometriosis recurrence with ART treatment and assures that no adverse effect of recurrence was seen on the ART Outcome. In patients with recurrence, where medical treatment fails or is contradicted or denied, A repeat surgery for recurrence can be offered to the patient If symptoms like dysmenorrhea or pelvic pain is a huge concern.

Sclerotherapy feasibility in programming, cost-effectiveness, and rapid recovery after the technique suggest that it can be considered the standard of care for minimally invasive interventions, like ethanol sclerotherapy of ovarian endometrioma who have completed family.

**Evidence gap:** A standard definition of "endometriosis-recurrence" should be framed and more research is needed particularly on the pre and postoperative medical treatment.

### Q2. How can we diagnose and manage extrapelvic endometriosis?

**Draft recommendation:**

*Imaging for diagnosing extrapelvic endometriosis*

- Transvaginal ultrasound (TVS) is a primary imaging tool. For extrapelvic locations, high-resolution transabdominal ultrasound is particularly useful for assessing bladder, ureters, and bowel involvement.
- Magnetic Resonance Imaging (MRI) is considered the gold standard for diagnosing extrapelvic endometriosis. MRI is particularly useful in detecting endometriotic lesions in atypical locations like the diaphragm, bowel, and nerves.
- Computed Tomography (CT) imaging is less commonly used for endometriosis due to its lower soft tissue resolution. It may help diagnose, exclude, or suggest the presence of a mass and define its extent and nature.
- Contrast CT improves the sensitivity and specificity (Gidwaney R, Badler RL et al., Hirata T, Koga K et al.). However, it can be helpful in emergency settings to evaluate complications such as bowel obstruction or urinary tract involvement.

**Summary of evidence:** Extrapelvic endometriosis (EPE) is a complex and challenging condition to diagnose due to its atypical presentation and diverse locations, including the gastrointestinal tract, urinary system, and thoracic cavity. Accurate diagnosis is crucial for effective management and improving patient outcomes. The diagnosis of extrapelvic endometriosis requires a combination of advanced imaging techniques, thorough clinical evaluation, and adherence to updated international guidelines.

*Location of extrapelvic endometriosis:*

*Abdominal wall endometriosis* is usually associated with gynecological procedures such as Caesarean section, laparoscopy, or abdominal hysterectomy. Scar endometriosis of Caesarean section is the most common abdominal wall endometriotic lesion and is mostly located at the site of the surgical incision. *Scar endometriosis* is estimated to occur in 0.03–1.5% of women after Caesarean delivery (Hirata T, Koga K et al.).

*Umbilical endometriosis* is rare, and the incidence is mostly 0.5–1.0% of all cases of endometriosis. Episiotomy endometriosis is quite rare and is estimated to occur in 0.01–0.06% of women after episiotomy (Hirata T, Koga K et al.).

*Thoracic endometriosis* is usually diagnosed based on clinical grounds. The symptoms are typically recurring in a cyclical pattern, occurring about 24 hours before and 72 hours after the onset of menstrual period (Rousset P, Rousset-Jablonski C et al.). Thoracic endometriosis syndrome (TES) presents in two forms, the pleural form with catamenial (menstruation) pneumothorax, non-catamenial endometriosis-related pneumothorax, catamenial hemothorax, and the pulmonary form with catamenial hemoptysis and lung nodules (Rousset P, Rousset-Jablonski C et al.). TES is the term used to refer to the various clinical and radiological manifestations resulting from the presence and cyclical changes of functional endometrial tissue in a thoracic structure (visceral or parietal pleura, lung parenchyma, airways, or diaphragm) (Rousset P, Rousset-Jablonski C et al.).

**Diagnostic modalities**

*Transvaginal ultrasound:* Transvaginal ultrasound (TVS) is a primary imaging tool. For extrapelvic locations, high-resolution transabdominal ultrasound is particularly useful for assessing bladder, ureters, and bowel involvement.

*Magnetic resonance imaging:* Magnetic Resonance Imaging is considered the gold standard for diagnosing extrapelvic endometriosis due to its superior soft tissue contrast and multiplanar capabilities. MRI is particularly useful in detecting endometriotic lesions in atypical locations like the diaphragm, bowel, and nerves. It provides detailed images of soft tissues, aiding in the detection of endometriotic lesions and mapping the extent of disease, which is crucial for preoperative planning.

*Computed tomography scans:* These are often used as complementary tools when other imaging modalities suggest extrapelvic disease involvement. Computed tomography (CT) and MRI may be used to diagnose or exclude alternative diagnoses in the anterior abdominal and pelvic wall, including hernia, abscess, hematoma from other causes, and other soft-tissue tumors (Hirata T, Koga K et al.).

*Collaborative efforts* among medical societies have led to more comprehensive diagnostic protocols, emphasizing non-invasive imaging and individualized patient care. As research continues to uncover new insights into the disease's etiology and progression, these guidelines will evolve, improving outcomes for women affected by this challenging condition.

**Management for extrapelvic endometriosis**

**Draft recommendation:**

- Treatment depends on the location. Surgical removal is the treatment of choice for abdominal extrapelvic endometriosis. Hormone treatment is an alternate option when surgical treatment is not possible. Hormone therapy can be offered for the treatment of thoracic endometriosis.

- A multidisciplinary team should be involved if surgery is indicated, involving a thoracic surgeon and/or other relevant specialists.
- Complete excision is the treatment of choice but if excision is not possible, long-term medical treatment is required (Andres MP, Arcoverde FVL et al.).
- The same principles of medical treatment for pelvic endometriosis apply for extragenital endometriosis also.
- For umbilical endometriosis surgical excision can be done but medical treatment may also be beneficial. Oral progestins, gonadotropin-releasing hormone agonists, and oral contraceptives can be used.
- For thoracic and diaphragmatic endometriosis, hormone therapy has been shown to be effective, but the recurrence rate is high.
- In recurrent pneumothorax or hemothorax, chemical pleurodesis, pleural abrasion or pleurectomy may be helpful.

**Summary of evidence:**

*Abdominal wall and perineal:* Complete excision of the nodule is done in case of abdominal wall and perineal endometriosis. Recurrence after excision may occur in a few cases.

*Umbilical:* Surgical excision of the lesion can be done but medical treatment may also be beneficial.

*Inguinal region:* A multidisciplinary approach is advised due to the proximity to neural structures and femoral vessels (Hirata T, Koga K et al.).

*Thoracic and diaphragmatic:* Hormone therapy (OCP or GnRH agonist) has been shown to be effective, but the recurrence rate is high.

In cases of *recurrent pneumothorax or hemothorax,* chemical pleurodesis, pleural abrasion or pleurectomy may be helpful (Gil Y, Tulandi T et al.). Lobectomy or segmentectomy is done for persistent hemoptysis due to parenchymal lesions (Gil Y, Tulandi T et al.).

If *catamenial pneumothorax is* due to diaphragmatic endometriosis, clinician should consider investigation and treatment of pelvic endometriosis. (Gil Y, Tulandi T et al.). In the case of catamenial pneumothorax when a patient does not want to undergo thoracic surgery or only incomplete resection is expected, a bilateral salpingo-oophorectomy (BSO) may be considered in absence of future fertility plans (Ciriaco P, Muriana P et al.).

According to recent meta-analysis by Ciriaco et al., on the treatment of thoracic endometriosis syndrome, video-assisted thoracoscopy (VATS) was the preferred surgical technique (Ciriaco P, Muriana P et al.). Recurrence of symptoms was documented in 27% of patients.

### Q3. How can we manage asymptomatic endometriosis?

**Draft recommendation:**

- Women should be informed and counselled about the incidental findings.
- Neither surgical treatment at time of surgery nor medical treatment are recommended for incidental finding of asymptomatic endometriosis *except* when associated with infertility.
- The further management of asymptomatic endometriosis should depend on the accuracy of diagnosis, age of the women, size of the mass, desire to preserve fertility and her psychological make-up.

**Summary of evidence:**

*Asymptomatic endometriosis* is peritoneal, ovarian, or deep endometriosis existing without any sign and symptoms of pain and/or infertility. It is found incidentally during surgery (sterilization, ovarian drilling for PCOS, appendectomy), examinations (e.g., fertility work-up, general gynecological examinations) and ultrasound for health check-ups.

The prevalence of asymptomatic endometriosis in the general population is not known but is said to be 3- 45 % in women undergoing laparoscopic tubal ligation surgeries (Gylfason JT et al., 2010).

Treatment of endometriosis is mainly based on overall symptoms. In asymptomatic women diagnosis and treatment are more challenging. Accurate diagnosis of asymptomatic endometriosis by non-invasive modalities is difficult to ascertain. Also, risk of asymptomatic minimal disease becoming symptomatic is low (Moen MH 2002).

No clinical trials are available to assess whether surgery or medical management are beneficial compared to expectant management. Surgical procedure—surgical excision or ablation are associated with surgical complications like adhesions and damage to adjacent anatomical structures. It is also difficult to recommend medical management without any evidence of progression of disease. Therefore, neither laparoscopic fulgrations at time of surgery nor medical treatment are recommended for incidental finding of asymptomatic endometriosis (ESHRE 2022).

Women should be informed and counselled about the findings and should be kept under long term follow up with repeated imaging every 3–6 months. This is to prevent the progression of disease and development of symptoms and to avoid a potential malignant transformation (ESHRE 2022).

Surgical management should be considered if there is a sudden enlargement in the cyst, symptoms such as pain and infertility occur, when malignancy cannot be ruled out, or if the women cannot come for follow-up regularly.

A recent prospective study reported that deep endometriosis could lead to detrusor overactivity. Hence urodynamic evaluation to assess bladder function in asymptomatic women could be correlated with the presence of deep endometriosis (Serati M 2013).

**Research gap:** Further randomized control trials (RCT) are recommended to determine the benefit of medical management, surgical management and long-term expectant management in cases of asymptomatic endometriosis.

### Q4. Is there a role of primary prevention of endometriosis?

**Draft recommendations:**

- Tailored early intervention strategies for high-risk individuals informed by familial predisposition and clinical risk assessment, could prove beneficial.
- *Risk factors:* Epidemiological data suggest that early menarche, shorter cycle length, long and heavy menstrual flow, lean body size and reduced gravidity/parity are associated with increased risk of developing endometriosis. Exposure to environmental pollutants, such as dioxins and polychlorinated biphenyls, do not draw a firm conclusion about the risk of developing endometriosis later in life. Nickel allergy seems to be a risk factor for endometriosis (Parazzani et al., 2017).
- Clinicians are encouraged to adopt a personalized approach, integrating lifestyle counseling and hormonal management based on individual patient profiles and risk assessments.
- Consider promoting a healthy lifestyle with regular physical activity and a balanced diet rich in fruits, vegetables, and omega-3 fatty acids as potential measures to mitigate endometriosis risk.
- While hormonal contraceptives and GnRH agonists are options for menstrual suppression, their efficacy for primary prevention remains uncertain.

**Summary of evidence:**

*Lifestyle modifications:* Endometriosis is a multifaceted condition influenced by genetic, hormonal, and environmental factors. Evidence supporting lifestyle modifications for preventing endometriosis is still evolving, with observational studies suggesting potential benefits of dietary adjustments and physical activity in regulating estrogen levels and potentially mitigating disease progression (Barnard ND et al., 2023).

*Diet:* Some studies suggest that a diet rich in fruits, vegetables, and omega-3 fatty acids may have protective effects. However, more research is needed to confirm these findings. Reducing dietary fat and increasing dietary fiber have been shown to reduce circulating estrogen concentrations, suggesting a potential benefit for individuals with endometriosis, as it is an estrogen-dependent disease. Meat consumption is associated with greater risk of developing endometriosis. Anti-inflammatory properties of plant-based diets may benefit women with endometriosis. Additionally, seaweed holds estrogen-modulating properties that have benefitted postmenopausal women and offers potential to reduce estradiol concentrations in pre-menopausal women. Supplementation of Vitamin D with vitamins C and E reduces endometriosis symptoms, compared with placebo. More randomized clinical trials are needed to elucidate the role of diet in endometriosis.

*Hormonal contraceptives and GnRH agonists:* These are commonly used to suppress menstruation, which may reduce the development of endometrial lesions, but definitive evidence on their effectiveness in primary prevention is lacking (Yu E et al., 2022, Christian M Becker et al., 2023). It is plausible that prolonged use of the OCP (continuous) and the LNG-IUD could potentially delay, minimize or even prevent the onset of symptomatic endometriosis. Regarding timing suppression, treatment should not be initiated before menarche to ensure proper onset of menarche and pubertal development. Suppression might be continued until the patient is willing to conceive. Nevertheless, a study revealed that women are not averse to the idea of eliminating menstruation; as many as 59% of women in the USA expressed a desire to eliminate their monthly periods (Christian M Becker et al., 2023).

*Genetic predisposition* plays a significant role, with women having a family history of endometriosis at increased risk (Fraser IS, et al., 2007). Identifying the targeted group for primary prevention is crucial; as only a small percentage (approximately 10%) of women eventually develop endometriosis within the general reproductive-age population, there is a need to identify those at greatest risk and implement preventive therapies that could potentially forestall or delay the onset of the disease process (Fraser IS et al., 2007).

*Public health initiatives* should prioritize raising awareness about endometriosis symptoms and promoting early diagnosis to optimize management strategies (Yu E et al., 2022).

Clinicians are encouraged to adopt a personalized approach, integrating lifestyle counseling and hormonal management based on individual patient profiles and risk assessments ((Fraser IS, et al., 2007).

### Q5. Is there any association between cancer and endometriosis?

**Draft recommendations:**

- Endometriosis is primarily a benign disease; malignant transformation has been reported rarely. The most common site of malignant development is the ovary.
- Endometriosis has been linked to an increased risk of ovarian cancer; particularly, endometriosis is associated with a greater risk of clear cell and endometrioid histotypes, equal to 3.4-fold and 2.3-fold, respectively (Kvaskoff et al.). However, the absolute risk is extremely low.

**Summary of evidence:**
Based on the meta-analysis, on association between endometriosis and prognosis of ovarian cancer by Peng Chen published in March 2022 included twenty-one studies involving 38641 patients were included. There were significant differences in overall survival and progression-free survival (PFS) between endometriosis-associated ovarian cancer (EAOC) and non-EAOC patients in the random-effects models.

Based on the meta-analysis and systematic review of endometriosis and cancer conducted by Martina et al., in February 2021. 49 population-based case-control and cohort studies were included. Cancer-specific analyses showed a positive association between endometriosis and ovarian cancer risk that was strongest for clear cell and endometrioid histotypes, although with significant evidence of both heterogeneity across studies and publication bias.

**Research gap:** Identification of shared genetic mechanism between endometriosis and gynecological cancers will open avenues for future disease management and treatment.

## BIBLIOGRAPHY

1. Andres MP, Arcoverde FVL, Souza CCC, et al. Extrapelvic endometriosis: a systematic review. J Minim Invasive Gynecol. 2020;27:373-89.
2. Andrist LC, Arias RD, Nucatola D, et al. Women's and providers' attitudes toward menstrual suppression with extended use of oral contraceptives. Contraception. 2004;70(5):359-63.
3. Barnard ND, Holtz DN, Schmidt N, et al. Nutrition in the prevention and treatment of endometriosis: a review. Front Nutr. 2023;10:1089891.
4. Becker CM, Bokor A, Heikinheimo O, et al. ESHRE guideline: endometriosis. Human Reprod Open. 2022:2:hoac009.
5. Chamie LP, Ribeiro D, Tiferes DA, et al. Atypical sites of deeply infiltrative endometriosis: clinical characteristics and imaging findings. Radiographics. 2018;38:309-28.
6. Chen P, Zhang CY. Association between endometriosis and prognosis of ovarian cancer: an updated meta-analysis. Front Oncol. 2022;12:732322.
7. Chiaffarino F, Cipriani S, Ricci E, et al. Histologic subtypes in endometriosis-associated ovarian cancer and ovarian cancer arising in endometriosis: a systematic review and meta-analysis. Reprod Sci. 2024;31(6):1642-50.
8. Fraser IS. The promise and reality of the intrauterine route for hormone delivery for prevention and therapy of gynecological disease. Contraception. 2007;75(6 Suppl):S112-7.
9. Gidwaney R, Badler RL, Yam BL, et al. Endometriosis of abdominal and pelvic wall scars: multimodality imaging findings, pathologic correlation, and radiologic mimics. Radiographics. 2012;32:2031-43.
10. Gil Y, Tulandi T. Diagnosis and treatment of catamenial pneumothorax: a systematic review. J Minim Invasive Gynecol. 2020;27(1):48-53.
11. Gylfason JT, Kristjansson KA, Sverrisdottir G, et al. Pelvic endometriosis diagnosed in an entire nation over 20 years. Am J Epidemiol. 2010;172:237-43.

12. Hirata T, Koga K, Kitade M, et al. A National Survey of Umbilical Endometriosis in Japan. J Minim Invasive Gynecol. 2020;27:80-7.
13. Joseph J, Reed CE, Sahn SA. Thoracic endometriosis. Recurrence following hysterectomy with bilateral salpingo-oophorectomy and successful treatment with talc pleurodesis. Chest. 1994;106:1894-6.
14. Kim SJ, Choi SH, Won S, et al. Cumulative Recurrence Rate and Risk Factors for Recurrent Abdominal Wall Endometriosis after Surgical Treatment in a Single Institution. Yonsei Med J. 2022;63(5):446-51.
15. Kvaskoff M, Mahamat-Saleh Y, Farland LV, et al. Endometriosis and cancer: a systematic review and meta-analysis. Hum Reprod Update. 2021;27(2):393-420.
16. Lee N, Min S, Won S, et al. The recurrence rate of ovarian endometrioma in women aged 40–49 years and impact of hormonal treatment after conservative surgery. Sci Rep. 2020;10(1):16461.
17. Li XY, Chao XP, Leng JH, et al. Risk factors for postoperative recurrence of ovarian endometriosis: long-term follow-up of 358 women. J Ovarian Res. 2019;12(1):79.
18. Ludovico M, Galati G, Mattei G, et al. Expectant, Medical, and Surgical Management of Ovarian Endometriomas. J Clin Med. 2023;12(5):1858.
19. Moen MH, Stokstad T. A long-term follow-up study of women with asymptomatic endometriosis diagnosed incidentally at sterilization. Fertil Steril. 2002;78:773-6.
20. Mortlock S, Corona RI, Kho PF, et al. A multi-level investigation of the genetic relationship between endometriosis and ovarian cancer histotypes. Cell Rep Med. 2022;3(3):100542.
21. Parazzini F, Esposito G, Tozzi L, et al. Epidemiology of endometriosis and its comorbidities. Eur J Obstet Gynecol Reprod Biol. 2017;209: 3-7.
22. Peng C, Huang Y, Zhou Y. Dydrogesterone in the treatment of endometriosis: evidence mapping and meta-analysis. Arch Gynecol Obstet. 2021;304(1):231-52.
23. RCOG. The initial management of chronic pelvic pain. Royal Coll Obstet Gynaecol. 2012;41:1-6.
24. Ronsini C, Iavarone I, Braca E, et al. The efficiency of sclerotherapy for the management of endometrioma: a systematic review and meta-analysis of clinical and fertility outcomes. Medicina (Kaunas). 2023;59(9):1643.
25. Rousset P, Rousset-Jablonski C, Alifano M, et al. Thoracic endometriosis syndrome: CT and MRI features. Clin Radiol. 2014;69:323-30.
26. Serati M, Cattoni E, Braga A, et al. Deep endometriosis and bladder and detrusor functions in women without urinary symptoms: a pilot study through an unexplored world. Fertil Steril. 2013;100:1332-6.
27. Simpson JL, Elias S, Malinak LR, et al. Heritable aspects of endometriosis. I. Genetic studies. Am J Obstet Gynecol. 1980;137(3):327-31.
28. Surrey ES. GnRH agonists in the treatment of symptomatic endometriosis: a review. F S Rep. 2022;4(2):40-5.
29. Vigueras Smith A, Cabrera R, Kondo W, et al. Diaphragmatic endometriosis minimally invasive treatment: a feasible and effective approach. J Obstet Gynaecol. 2020:1-11.
30. Yarmish G, Sala E, Goldman DA, et al. Abdominal wall endometriosis: differentiation from other masses using CT features. Abdom Radiol (NY). 2017;42:1517-23.
31. Ye J, Peng H, Huang X, et al. The association between endometriosis and risk of endometrial cancer and breast cancer: a meta-analysis. BMC Womens Health. 2022;22(1):455.